The Orthopaedically Handicapped Child

National Children's Bureau Bibliographies

6

The Orthopaedically Handicapped Child

Rosemary Dinnage

NFER-NELSON

Published by the NFER-NELSON Publishing Company Ltd.,
Darville House, 2 Oxford Road East,
Windsor, Berkshire SL4 1DF, England

and in the United States of America by

NFER-NELSON, 242 Cherry Street, Philadelphia, PA 19106–1906.
Tel: (215) 238 0939. Telex: 244489.

First Published 1986
© 1986 National Children's Bureau

Library of Congress Cataloging in Publication data
Dinnage, Rosemary.
  The orthopaedically handicapped child.

  Updated version of: The orthopaedically handicapped child / Doria
Pilling. 1972.
  Includes index.
  1. Pediatric orthopedia – Abstracts. I. Pilling, Doria. Orthopaedically
handicapped child. II. Title. [DNLM: 1. Handicapped – abstracts. 2.
Orthopedics – in infancy & childhood – abstracts. 3. Rehabilitation –
abstracts ZWS 270 D585o]
RD732.3.C48D55   1986   362.4'088054   86–5260
ISBN 0–7005–1021–4

Photoset by David John (Services) Ltd., Maidenhead

Printed in Great Britain by Henry Ling Ltd., at the Dorset Press, Dorchester, Dorset

ISBN 0–7005–1021–4
Code 8207 02 1

Contents

Acknowledgements

Thanks are due first to the Department of Health and Social Security whose grant made this review possible.

The National Children's Bureau's librarians, Ian Vallender and Biddy Cunnell, provided invaluable help in searching for references and obtaining books and photocopies. The librarian of the Tavistock Centre, Margaret Walker, was most helpful in providing further references by means of a computer scan.

The Muscular Dystrophy Group of Great Britain kindly supplied a booklist.

Finally, Doria Pilling, author of these booklets in their first edition, is not only responsible for part of the contents but has advised on the updated version.

Introduction

In 1972–73 the National Children's Bureau published a series of concise research review booklets on childhood handicaps. Non-medical studies were summarized, and a brief overview added. In the years since, a great deal of further research and discussion has been published, and the Bureau felt it would be useful to have updated versions. The new booklets, therefore, contain material that was in the originals, together with more recent entries; and the reviews prefacing the annotated bibliographies have been rewritten.

The present booklet summarizes research literature on children with orthopaedic handicaps – the term being used to cover a wide variety of conditions which impair the functioning of muscles, bones or joints and which may be due to congenital abnormalities or acquired through accident, infection or disease. Two categories that were included in the earlier version – post-polio impairment and thalidomide deformities – have been excluded as no longer of current importance. There has been space available to include a fuller section on attitudes to handicap, and in Section IV a number of articles about integrated schooling.

There are difficulties in any categorization of handicap. In general, the physical disabilities included here do not involve any brain abnormality. There is evidence, though, that in progressive muscular dystrophy of the Duchenne type (a degenerative disorder of the muscle probably due to a metabolic defect) there is an increased incidence of mental retardation that cannot be accounted for solely by educational limitations or emotional factors. While, then, there may be brain involvement the nature of this is unknown. Nevertheless muscular dystrophy is primarily a disease of muscle and it appears most satisfactory to include it with the orthopaedic handicaps – a heterogeneous grouping, in any case. Cerebral palsy and spina bifida each form the subject of another booklet; all these booklets will be most useful if read together.

SECTION I
Attitudes to Disability

This is an area in which there has been a great deal of research interest, particularly in America. The attitudes that others have towards him is obviously a crucial factor in a child's social and emotional adjustment. If children with orthopaedic handicaps are viewed unfavourably, then this may be a more important factor in their development than the actual physical limitations.

Research on attitudes to the handicap has not produced a definitive conclusion. Many studies have started from the position that attitudes are negative. The most frequently used measure has been the Attitude Towards Disabled Persons scale (Yuker *et al.*, 1966). This measures attitudes to disabled people as a group and sums up the respondent's attitude in a single score. The scale has both inspired research and attracted criticism. It does not differentiate between disabilities, nor does it take into account the complexity of attitudes towards the disabled (Siller and Chipman, 1964). Attitudes may vary, then, with the type of disability, the situation and characteristics of the non-handicapped person.

A number of studies have tried to find a preference order for people with various types of disabilities (Jones *et al.*, 1966; Shears and Jensema, 1969; Tringo, 1970), using some version of the social distance technique (subjects are asked the closest relationship they would allow with a person with a particular type of disability). Reasonably consistent results have been found using varied samples – high school and college students and adults. In most situations – having the disabled person as a friend, co-worker, playmate for a child – those with orthopaedic conditions are viewed favourably compared with those having sensory or neurological abnormalities. A similar hierarchy was found in a study (Barsch, 1964) in which a large number of adults, including parents of handicapped and non-handicapped children, rated disabilities according to their severity for a child. When subjects were asked about their willingness to marry a disabled person, however, the crippled dropped in acceptability, indicating that there are different determinants of attitudes here.

Research in which the subject is actually placed in a face-to-face situation with an apparently orthopaedically handicapped person has confirmed the complexity of attitudes (Kleck *et al.*, 1966; Farina *et al.*, 1968). Although the non-handicapped subjects (high school or college students) were more inhibited with a person they thought to be physically handicapped than with a normal person in the first study, both studies found the subjects

1

being 'kind' to the apparently handicapped.

A series of studies by Richardson and his colleagues has dealt specifically with the attitudes of children to other children with various orthopaedic and cosmetic disabilities (Richardson *et al.,* 1961; Richardson, 1970). A picture of a non-handicapped child was almost universally preferred to pictures of children with various handicaps. There was also considerable uniformity in preference for specific types of handicaps. The most recent study investigates the relationship between attitudes and actual behaviour (Richardson, 1971). While judgements about handicapped children depended on prejudices at first encounters, they were modified later, when the personal qualities of the handicapped child became known. Much may depend, though, on the atmosphere provided by adults; the study took place at a summer camp where friendships between all children were encouraged, regardless of handicaps.

The most recent research included here tends to concentrate on the question of modifying children's attitudes to their handicapped peers early on (though Altman (1981) calls for less research on children and more on influential adults such as employers). In the background of this research on young children's attitudes is the question of integrating schooling for handicapped and non-handicapped; the recurrent theme is that it is actual contact with children with varied handicaps which leads to more spontaneous and unprejudiced attitudes.

Rapier and his colleagues (1972) asked children about their attitudes to orthopaedically handicapped peers before and after a year of integrated schooling; on the whole, unrealistic stereotypes had changed for the better. Three projects concentrate on specific programmes for changing attitudes. Donaldson and Martinson (1977) worked with university students, and tried to encourage contact with the world of the handicapped by means of discussion groups; live and taped discussions with handicapped students changed the subjects' attitudes towards them. Handlers' and Austin's (1980) subjects were high school pupils, taking a course on the problems of handicap. The great majority reported a swing towards more sympathetic attitudes after the course, and rated the most valuable part of it the discussion with a blind person. Rosenbaum and Armstrong (1984) conducted an ingenious experiment in which normal children acted as 'buddies' to a handicapped child for a time. Again, there was a swing towards positive attitudes. All these projects reinforce the suggestion that contact with handicapped children or persons tends to dispel negative preconceptions.

Attitudes towards a significantly different group are enormously complex; there is a confusion of fears and fantasies, aversion and sympathy, which it is hard to tap by pencil-and-paper tests. It does, at any rate, seem that actual contact with handicap goes some way towards dispelling ignorance and prejudice.

Section I: *Attitudes to Disability*

RICHARDSON,
S.A., GOODMAN,
N., HASTORF,
A.H., and
DORNBUSCH,
S.M.
(1961)
*American
Sociological
Review*, 26, 2,
241–7.

Cultural uniformity in reaction to physical disabilities

Groups of 10- to 11-year-old children from diverse backgrounds were found to rank six pictures of children with visible handicaps in the same order of preference. Within each group there was significant agreement on ranking. The order of preference was: (1) no handicap; (2) crutches and brace; (3) wheelchair; (4) left hand missing; (5) facial disfigurement; and (6) an obese child. Sex, race, socioeconomic status, presence of physical handicap or experience with handicapped children did not affect the order. Compared with the boys, though, the girls liked the children with social impairments (obesity and facial disfigurement) less. The boys liked the children with disabilities affecting physical activity less than did the girls. Explanations for the order of preference are discussed.

BILLINGS, H.K.
(1963)
*Journal of
Experimental
Education*, 31,
381–7.

An exploratory study of the attitudes of non-crippled children toward crippled children in three selected elementary schools

School children's attitudes towards their crippled peers were explored by means of projective tests. Fifty-four children from three grades in three schools had to complete stories and sentences about normal and crippled children and their responses were assessed on a four-point scale. Teachers' ratings of the social adjustment of each child were obtained. Attitudes towards crippled schoolmates were more unfavourable than towards the normal and the unfavourable attitudes increased with age (from 6.5 to 11.8 years). Contrary to prediction, there was a positive relation between good adjustment and greater prejudice.

CENTERS, L. and
CENTERS, R.
(1963a)
*Journal of Social
Psychology*, 61, 1,
127–32.

Peer group attitudes toward the amputee child

Normal children (aged five to 12 years from 28 classes) were found to show more rejecting attitudes towards classmates with upper extremity amputations than to their non-handicapped classmates. An amputee child was named as the saddest child in the class eight times as often as a non-handicapped child.

GOFFMAN, E.
(1963)
Engelwood Cliffs:
Prentice-Hall Inc.
Also published by
Penguin Books,
Harmondsworth,
Middlesex. 1968.

Stigma. Notes on the management of spoiled identity

A penetrating sociological discussion of the situation and social role of the individual with handicap or abnormality of any kind. Autobiographical and case material is extensively quoted.

BARSCH, R.M.
(1964)
*American Journal
of Public Health,*
54, 9, 1560–7.

The handicapped ranking scale among parents of handicapped children

Close agreement about the severity in childhood of ten handicapping conditions was found among 2375 subjects (parents of handicapped and non-handicapped children, teachers, nurses and other hospital staff). Cerebral palsy was seen as the severest handicap, followed by mental retardation, mental illness, brain injury, blindness, epilepsy, deafness, polio, heart trouble and diabetes. Those who were in close contact with a particular disability tended to see it as being relatively less severe.

SILLER, J. and
CHIPMAN, A.
(1964)
*Educational and
Psychological
Measurement,*
24, 4, 831–40.

Factorial structure and correlates of the Attitudes Toward Disabled Persons scale

An examination of the most widely used instrument for measuring attitudes towards the disabled, the Attitudes Towards Disabled Persons scale. The authors suggest that the ATDP measures the attitude that the handicapped 'differ in certain ways from the general population' rather than the 'degree of acceptance of the handicapped'. They believe that 'acceptance' of the handicapped is compatible with perceiving them as different in some ways from the physically normal population. Attitudes towards the disabled are multidimensional and cannot be expressed in a single score as the ATDP attempts to do.

JONES, R.L.,
GOTTFRIED,
N.W., and
OWENS, A.
(1966)
*Exceptional
Children,* 32, 8,
551–6.

The social distance of the exceptional: a study at the high school level

186 high school students were asked to compare the acceptability of ten types of handicapped person, the average and the gifted, in a number of different social situations. In most situations the average and gifted were the most acceptable and the mentally retarded the least. The acceptability of the other handicaps varied

with the situation, but those with mild handicaps were placed highest. The crippled and the chronically ill were usually placed below this group and above the blind, deaf, emotionally disturbed and delinquent. In the situation 'I would accept this person as close kin by marrige', though, the acceptability of the crippled dropped much lower.

KLECK, R., ONI, H., and HASTORF, A.H. (1966) *Human Relations,* 19, 4, 425–36.

The effects of physical deviance upon face-to-face interaction

Two experiments were conducted to explore the hypothesis that a normal person meeting a physically handicapped person for the first time in a face-to-face situation will behave in a stereotyped, inhibited and over-controlled manner. An interview situation was used in both experiments. In half of the interviews in each experiment the interviewer appeared to be physically disabled. As predicted, when faced with a physically disabled interviewer, subjects (college students in the first experiment and high school juniors in the second) showed less variability in their behaviour as a group than when the interviewer was not disabled; they distorted their replies so as to be 'kind' to the interviewer; and the interview ended sooner.

YUKER, H.E., BLOCK, J.R., and YOUNG, J.H. (1966 and 1970) Albertson, New York, 1NA MEND Institute at Human Resources Center.

The Measurement of Attitudes Towards Disabled Persons

Description of the Attitudes Toward Disabled Persons Scale (ATDP), devised by the authors, and comprehensive review of research on attitudes towards the disabled using this and other measures. The ATDP attempts to measure attitudes towards the disabled in general, rather than towards specific disabilities. Results show the extent to which the respondent perceives the disabled as being different from the non-disabled. The authors believe that being 'different' can be interpreted as a negative reaction, suggesting inferiority. Tentative conclusions about acceptance of the disabled from the research review are that: (1) there is a curvilinear relationship with education – attitudes becoming less favourable through school but reversing at high school and college levels; (2) females have more favourable attitudes than males; (3) those with more positive self-concepts are more accepting; (4) there is no definite evidence as to whether the ATDP reflects self-concept when used with disabled respondents; (5) there is a positive relationship with the acceptance of others who are 'different', e.g. minority ethnic groups; (6) increased contact with the disabled results in more favourable responses – possible exceptions are contact in a medical or rehabilitation setting or with a disabled sibling.

5

FEINBERG, L.B.
(1967)
*Personnel and
Guidance Journal,*
46, 4, 375–81.

Social desirability and attitudes toward the disabled

Attempts to investigate the attitudes of the non-disabled towards the disabled have produced contradictory findings. Previous studies have not taken into account the need of the non-disabled person to be seen in a socially desirable light – and publicity campaigns in recent years have suggested that it is socially desirable to help the handicapped. The present study administered three attitude-toward-disability scales to 280 university students. As predicted, those who had high social desirability needs responded with significantly more favourable attitudes towards the disabled than did those with low social desirability needs.

JAFFE, J.
(1967)
*Personnel and
Guidance Journal,*
45, 6, 557–60.

'What's in a name' – attitudes toward disabled persons

Many studies of attitudes towards the disabled use a term or 'label' such as 'cripple' to elicit attitudes. This study compared the responses of high school students to three such 'labels' (amputees, mentally retarded, former mental patients) with the responses of other students to written sketches of persons, described as having one of these disabilities. For all three disabilities attitudes were more favourable to the sketch person than to the 'label'. Attitudes towards the disabled may not be as negative as some studies using 'labels' suggest.

CHIGIER, E. and
CHIGIER, M.
(1968)
*Journal of Health
and Social
Behaviour,* 9, 4,
310–7.

Attitudes to disability of children in the multi-cultural society of Israel

Eleven groups of Israeli children, of diverse cultural background, degrees of religious orthodoxy and socioeconomic level, were shown the six pictures which had been used in American studies to determine the order of preference for various handicaps (see Richardson *et al.*, 1961). Eight of the groups, all from lower-class neighbourhoods but with varied cultural backgrounds, had the same preference order as lower-class American Jewish children, preferring cosmetic to physical handicaps. Two of the groups, from middle class areas, showed the American normative pattern, preferring physical to cosmetic handicaps. Contrary to the American studies the findings suggest that socioeconomic status may be an important determinant of attitudes towards the handicapped.

FARINA, A.,
SHERMAN, M.,
and
ALLEN, J.G.
(1968)
*Journal of
Abnormal
Psychology*, 73, 6,
590–3.

Role of physical abnormalities in interpersonal perception and behaviour

Goffman (1963) has argued that all deviations from normality lead to unfavourable reactions in relationships between the deviant and the normal. The authors of this study suggest that the behaviour of the non-handicapped is more complex, perception of another as abnormal sometimes leading to sympathetic treatment. Sixty male university students took part in an experiment in which each had to teach another subject, who was apparently either an amputee or slightly crippled, a pattern of responses, administering an electric shock to the learner when he made the wrong choice. Duration of shocks was shorter for the severely crippled subject, showing that in this situation he was more favourably treated.

JAFFE, J.
(1968)
*Dissertation
Abstracts*, 26, 2,
1119.

Attitudes of adolescents toward persons with disabilities

The attitudes of 477 high school students towards people with different types of disability were determined by their evaluations of a sketch person. Subjects were divided randomly into four groups and told that the sketch person was an amputee, mentally retarded, a former mental patient or no disability was mentioned. Contrary to expectations the amputee was evaluated the most favourably. It appears that when the disabled can be seen to function adequately attitudes towards them may be favourable.

CONINE, T.A.
(1969)
*Journal of School
Health*, 39, 4,
278–81.

Acceptance or rejection of disabled persons by teachers

Teachers in a midwestern city (half of a randomly selected sample of 1000 responded to the questionnaire) showed a degree of acceptance of the disabled similar to that of the general public (as measured by the Attitudes Toward Disabled Persons scale). Sex was the only variable significantly affecting attitudes, women teachers being more favourable to the disabled than men. The author points out the importance of changing teachers' attitudes if those of the public are to be changed.

McDANIEL, J.W.
(1969)
Chapter II in
*Physical Disability
and Human
Behaviour.*
Oxford:
Pergamon Press,
pp. 17–47.

Attitudes and disability

A review of research on attitudes to the disabled. Some important conclusions are: there is no universal stereotype for the physically disabled; attitudes towards disabilities may be more negative than attitudes to the disabled; prejudice against the disabled is associated with prejudice against all minorities; the degree of acceptance of the disabled by the non-disabled is related to age, sex, and possibly education and sophistication; further research is needed on the relationship between a person's satisfaction with his own body and his attitude to the disabled.

SHEARS, L.M. and
JENSEMA, C.J.
(1969)
*Exceptional
Children,* 36, 2,
91–6.

Social acceptability of anomalous persons

Ninety-four adult subjects were asked to rank 10 types of physically handicapped or socially deviant person according to their acceptability in various social situations. Acceptance of the disabled decreased gradually as the closeness of the social relationship increased. The ordering of preferences for the various disabilities was the same in most of the situations. Those with a visible disability (e.g. the amputee or blind) were most acceptable; those whose condition was associated with stigma (the mentally ill, retarded or homosexual) were least acceptable, while those with communication problems formed an intermediary group. Acceptability of a condition in a marriage partner or as a self-affliction showed some changes in rank order, suggesting that different factors are relevant here.

RICHARDSON,
S.A.
(1970)
*Journal of Health
and Social
Behaviour,* 2, 3,
207–14.

Age and sex differences in values toward physical handicaps

Using the picture ranking method (see Richardson *et al.*, 1961) attitudes towards various handicaps were studied in children at various age levels between five and 18 and in their parents. With increasing age the pictures of children with cosmetic handicaps (left hand missing and facial disfigurement) became less liked and those with functional handicaps (leg brace and crutches and wheelchair) became more liked. In general, as they became older the children's preferences became more like those of their parents. It seems that children do not learn values towards handicap directly from their parents. At early ages differences in overall appearance may be the chief cause of anxiety, while at later ages impairments take on social meanings.

TRINGO, J.L.
(1970)
*Journal of Special
Education*, 4, 3,
295–306.

The hierarchy of preference toward disability groups

Six groups of subjects (high school, college and graduate students and rehabilitation workers) were asked to indicate the closest relationship they would allow to a person in each of 21 disability groups. The order of preference for the disabilities was very similar for all the groups. As in other studies, the physically disabled were the most acceptable, followed by the sensory disabled, with the brain-injured least acceptable. The high school students were considerably less accepting than the other groups. Women in all the groups were more accepting than men.

LAZAR, A.L.,
GENSLEY, J.T.,
and ORPET, R.E.
(1971)
*Exceptional
Children*, 37, 8,
600–2.

Changing attitudes of young mentally gifted children toward handicapped persons

After a four-week instructional programme aimed at creating more understanding of the handicapped, 23 eight-year-old mentally gifted (IQs 123 plus) children showed more favourable attitudes to the disabled (as measured by the Attitudes Toward Disabled Persons scale) than before.

RICHARDSON,
S.A.
(1971)
*Journal of Health
and Social
Behaviour*, 12, 3,
253–8.

Children's values and friendships: a study of physical disability

This study explores the relationship between children's attitudes to other children with various physical disabilities, as shown in the picture ranking test and their actual behaviour as seen in friendship choices. Subjects were handicapped and non-handicapped, 9- to 13-year-old, lower-class children at a New York summer camp. Findings suggested that for the non-handicapped children attitudes were an important influence at first, choices having to be made mainly on appearance. Later, other children were judged by their personal qualities rather than by their handicap. The pattern was different for the handicapped children, who appeared initially to try to take advantage of the camp philosophy of integration and choose non-handicapped friends but later tended to choose handicapped friends as they felt the other children expected.

RAPIER, J.,
ADELSON, R.,
CAREY, R., and
CROKE, K.
(1972)
*Exceptional
Children,* 39, 3,
219–23.

Changes in children's attitudes towards the physically handicapped

From a school in California incorporating a unit for the orthopaedically handicapped, 152 children aged 8 to 11 were asked about their attitudes to the handicapped before and after a year of integrated schooling. Even before integration their attitudes were quite positive, but they changed in terms of seeing the handicapped children as not so weak and helpless as they had thought. Before integration there were sex differences in attitudes, but these disappeared after integration. Integrated schooling is valuable in changing children's negative stereotypes of handicap.

DIXON, J.K.
(1977)
*Journal of Chronic
Disease,* 30,
307–22.

Coping with prejudice: attitudes of handicapped persons towards the handicapped

An exploration of the amount of prejudice that handicapped people feel towards other handicapped people, compared to that felt by the able-bodied. It was found that a distinction should be made between relatively visible handicaps and relatively invisible ones. People with amputation, spinal injury and stroke (highly visible) had positive attitudes, but arthritics and emotionally disturbed people did not. These results suggest that promoting contacts between people with similar handicaps would only work well for those with the more visible handicaps.

DONALDSON, J.
and MARTINSON,
M.C.
(1977)
*Exceptional
Children,* 43, 6,
337–41.

Modifying attitudes towards physically disabled persons

Subjects were 120 non-disabled university students of both sexes, assigned to four experimental groups. A discussion was held with six visibly handicapped young people (cerebral palsy, blindness, etc.). One group of subjects sat in on a discussion with these people about their lives; one group saw a video of the discussion; one group heard a tape of it; one group did none of these things. All subjects filled in an 'Attitude Toward Disabled Persons Scale' afterwards. Results suggest that both a live and a videotaped discussion were effective in changing students' attitudes towards the disabled. There were no significant differences between male and female students' reactions. The use of such a videotape in education is discussed.

WEINBERG, N.
(1978)
*Rehabilitation
Counselling
Bulletin*, 21, 3,
183–9.

Preschool children's perceptions of orthopedic disability

Children of three, four and five were tested on their understanding of orthopaedic handicap. On the first experiment they were divided into two groups; half were shown a photograph of an able-bodied child and half of a child in a wheelchair. They were asked if they would like to play with the child, whether the child could run, sing and colour, and whether teacher and parents would want them to play with the handicapped children. They were then asked questions to determine whether they understood the disability involved. It was clear that understanding increased dramatically after three years of age. No differences were found at any age on the questions about liking, parental approval and the handicapped child's abilities.

On the second experiment another group of three- to five-year-olds were shown similar pictures and asked which of the two children they would rather play with. They were again asked questions to test their understanding of disability; and again, understanding seemed to come by four or five years. 73 per cent of the children preferred the able-bodied child as a playmate, the percentage rising with age. No sex differences were found in either experiment. The findings suggest that the attitudes of young children are flexible, as they only showed preference for the able-bodied when specifically asked to choose. Education about disability should evidently be started early.

HANDLERS, A.
and AUSTIN, K.
(1980)
*Exceptional
Children*, 47, 3,
228–9.

Improving attitudes of high school students towards their handicapped peers

Description of an experimental eight-week educational programme to enable high school students to become more knowledgeable about handicapped people and to ease the mainstreaming of handicapped children into class. The young people discussed terminology and laws; researched and reported on specific disabilities; watched a film about the handicapped; tried out simulation activities to experience what handicaps felt like; and talked to a blind student. Afterwards, 82 per cent said they felt that their attitudes had become more positive and accepting. A majority rated direct contact with the handicapped person as the most effective part of the scheme. The experiment was considered a success and was adopted for young people taking the sociology course.

ALTMAN, B.M.
(1981)
Social Problems,
28, 3, 321–37.

Studies of attitudes towards the handicapped: the need for a new direction

A review article of studies published over the past 25 years, with nearly 100 references. It is suggested that more research should be done on adult attitudes rather than children's, and especially those of people in positions of influence, such as employers, bank managers and police. The effect of educational 'mainstreaming' of handicapped children should be investigated. Attitudes are complex and multidimensional and future research should take account of this.

ROSENBAUM,
P.L.
and ARMSTRONG,
R.W.
(1984)
Paper presented at
annual convention
of the American
Psychological
Association in
Toronto, Canada.

Changing children's attitudes towards disabled peers: randomized controlled trials of buddy and educational programs

An account of three studies in changing children's attitudes carried out in Canada. In the first, children in grades 5 to 8 were asked if they would be a 'buddy' to a handicapped child; over half agreed. Their attitudes to handicap were first tested on a specially constructed questionnaire; then 42 children were randomly chosen and paired with a handicapped child for weekly non-academic activities for three months. The handicapped children were quite severely disabled, mainly by cerebral palsy or spina bifida. At the end of the three months, the 42 children, together with a control group who had not been 'buddies', were tested again on their attitudes. The 'buddies' had significantly more positive attitudes than the control group.

The second study used a puppet show relating to various handicaps. This was shown to schoolchildren once a week for ten weeks. Some children acted as 'buddies', some were 'buddies' and also saw the puppet programmes, and some were involved in neither activity. Although the attitude scores of the 'buddies' improved, those of the children who both acted as 'buddies' and also saw the puppet shows did not; it is suggested that the two programmes were not compatible with one another. The third study used only the puppet shows, and found that they had no effect on attitudes. The authors recommend extension of the 'buddy' type of experiment, but point out that only the children who had consented to it were involved. It would be valuable to know what the impact would be on children who refuse.

SECTION II
Emotional and Social Adjustment

Two important research studies have tended to find only slightly higher or the same rate of emotional disorder among physically handicapped children without brain disorders (including a high proportion with orthopaedic handicaps) as among the normal child population (Graham and Rutter, 1970; Anderson, 1973 (see Section IV)). Anderson was surveying a group of disabled schoolchildren attending ordinary schools; Graham and Rutter's study was of all the physically handicapped aged 10 to 12 on the Isle of Wight. Neither of these studies are strictly confined to orthopaedic handicaps, and neither deal with adolescents, who may well face more maladjustment than younger children.

There is no study, therefore, that comes up with a final answer about the emotional adjustment of the orthopaedically handicapped as a group – and the group is really too disparate for such an answer to be found. Pless and Pinkerton (1975) and Fox (1977) discuss the particular problems associated with physical handicap: restraint on mobility, isolation from peer group activities, confusion about the nature of the disability, difficulties in finding a role and an identity. Schechter (1961) suggests that there may often be denial, depression and a tendency to see the handicap as some sort of punishment. Volpe's (1976) study emphasizes the passivity characterizing children who have to rely on others for so much of their care.

There is a certain amount of research on specific disabilities. Seven papers on juvenile rheumatoid arthritis are included here. This disease has been associated with psychosomatic stresses, and some of the papers give support to the hypothesis. Rimon *et al.* (1977) studied a sample in Finland and found that 39 per cent of the children had suffered from an emotional disturbance before the disease started, and in 37 per cent there seemed to be a correlation between life stress and the onset of the illness. Henoch *et al.* (1978) found a much higher than average proportion of deaths, divorces and adoptions in the backgrounds of the patients they studied. There may also, however, be a genetic predisposition, and Rimon and his colleagues propose two groups, one with such a predisposition for whom stress is less important and one for whom onset is in fact linked with stress. McAnarney *et al.* (1974) and Wilkinson (1981) studied groups of children and adolescents respectively, and found a good deal of maladjustment, anxiety and depression among them. In McAnarney's sample the *less* handicapped children had the most maladjustment; he suggests that their role and their capabilities were less clearly defined than those of the severely handicapped.

Scoliosis has also attracted a certain amount of research interest. Here findings vary, Gratz and Papalia-Finlay (1984) finding the wearing of a brace well tolerated, and Schatzinger *et al.* (1977) finding that a large number of girls reacted badly to the brace and to surgery. Bengtsson *et al.* (1974), studying adult women with scoliosis in Scandinavia, concluded that under a facade of adjustment there was a great deal of insecurity.

Muscular dystrophy is in rather a special category, because of its prognosis. The main research interest has been in intellectual development (see Section IV), but some papers are included on emotional adjustment. Two studies used projective drawings to assess this (Siegel and Kornfeld, 1980; Pope-Grattan *et al.,* 1976); dependence, immaturity, and insecurity were their main findings. Sherwin and McCully (1961) describe the various means that boys with this illness use for coping with it. Adler (1973) describes a specially supportive programme for them which he feels might usefully be adopted.

KIMMEL, J.
(1959)
*Dissertation
Abstracts*, 19,
3023.

A comparison of children with congenital and acquired orthopaedic handicaps on certain personality characteristics

Fifteen 10- to 16-year-old children with congenital orthopaedic disabilities and 15 children with orthopaedic disabilities acquired after the age of five years were given two projective tests. The two groups were matched for age, sex, intelligence and severity of handicap. Children with acquired handicaps were found to have greater confidence and more esteem for their bodies and could cope more adequately with anxiety than the children with congenital disabilities. The two groups did not differ in family, school or social adjustment, or in attitude to the handicap or rehabilitation, according to their casework reports.

SCHECHTER,
M.D.
(1961)
*Archives of
General
Psychiatry*, 4, 3,
247–53.

The orthopaedically handicapped child. Emotional reactions

After four years' observation of children with acquired or congenital disabilities, in an orthopaedic hospital, the author concludes that there is no common personality pattern. Some similarities in reactions, though, do occur: denial of disability; seeing the illness as a punishment for misdeeds; depression; fear of leaving the hospital and of contact with those outside; hopelessness about the future; use of the deformity as a means of communication with others. Explanations are discussed for the lack of suicides or psychotic reactions, despite the severity of the symptoms.

SHERWIN, A.C.
and McCULLY,
R.S.
(1961)
*Journal of
Chronic Disease*,
13, 59–68.

Reactions observed in boys of various ages (ten to fourteen) to a crippling, progressive, and fatal illness (muscular dystrophy)

Fifteen boys with muscular dystrophy, attending a special day school, were observed over a one- to three-year period and given psychiatric and psychological evaluations. Although there was a relative absence of serious emotional illness and little overt anxiety about the disease, projective tests showed it to be an ever present stress. Attitudes to the disease showed rapid shifts from acceptance to denial, and fluctuation of attitudes characterized the children's behaviour in general. There was an excessive reliance on fantasy as a source of satisfaction. All the children had a strong motivation towards accomplishing tasks involving motor ability as well as possible. They had difficulty in relationships with others.

CENTERS, L. and
CENTERS, R.
(1963b)
*Journal of
Projective
Techniques and
Personality
Assessment*, 27, 2,
158–65.

A comparison of the body images of amputee and non-amputee children as revealed in figure drawings

The majority of a sample of 26 children, aged five to 12 years, with upper extremity amputations were found to be realistic about themselves (self-portraits showed a limb missing or prosthetic device), without undue conflict (the self-portraits showed only the same prevalence of factors supposed to be indicative of conflict and anxiety as did those of non-handicapped children), and aware of their difference from others (their portraits of 'a person' were indistinguishable from those of normal children). Nevertheless eight of the amputees drew themselves with two arms and this needs explanation.

GINGRAS, G. *et al.*
(1964)
*Canadian Medical
Association
Journal*, 91,
115–19.

Congenital anomalies of the limbs, Part II. Psychological and educational aspects

Forty-one children and adults with congenital limb deformities, who had attended the Montreal Rehabilitation Institute over the previous ten years, were assessed by a psychiatrist and a psychologist. Half of the parents were also interviewed. All but five of the subjects had normal intelligence or above. All except one of the school-age children attended ordinary schools. Only one child had a major emotional disorder. Conflicts which did occur were the same as those in normal children but were intensified by the physical anomaly. Parental acceptance was an important factor in the children's adjustment to their handicap and the wearing of prostheses. Psychotherapeutic help for the mother as soon as possible after the birth of a deformed child is recommended.

SCHORER, C.E.
(1964)
*Psychosomatic
Medicine*, 26, 1,
5–13.

Muscular dystrophy and the mind

An investigation of 28 males, aged five to 28 years, suffering from muscular dystrophy, by means of a psychiatric interview, human figure drawings and the Bender Gestalt test, supported the hypothesis that deprivation of motor experiences from an early age can have deforming effects on mental development. Early recognition of the defect and the use of compensatory measures might help the child to reach the best possible adjustment.

SMITS, S.J.
(1964)
*Dissertation
Abstracts*, 25, 2,
1324–5.

Reactions of self and others to the obviousness and severity of physical disability

Among 200 physically disabled adolescents attending ordinary schools in the St. Louis area, those with mild disabilities had higher self-concept scores than those with severe disabilities. Severely disabled girls had the lowest self-acceptance scores. On a sociometric test, the physically disabled, as a group, were rated lower by their classmates than the non-disabled.

BROOKS, M.B.
and SHAPERMAN,
J.
(1965)
*American Journal
of Occupational
Therapy*, 9, 6,
329–33.

Infant prosthetic fitting. A study of results

In a study of 68 children with congenital unilateral upper extremity deficiencies, fitting with a prosthesis before the age of two years was more successful than fitting between two and five years of age. The most important factor in acceptance of the prosthesis was the ability of parents to communicate with the child and with the professional personnel.

CLEVELAND,
S.E.,
REITMAN, E.E.,
and BREWER, E.J.
Jr.
(1965)
*Arthritis and
Rheumatism*, 8,
1152–8.

Psychological factors in juvenile rheumatoid arthritis

Thirty arthritic children, aged 6.5 to 16 years, and 25 asthmatic children, comparable in age, duration of illness and socio-economic level, were administered a number of psychological tests. Mothers of the arthritic children were also interviewed and given tests. As in previous studies with adults, the arthritic children appeared to have been more active than average before their illness. Unlike the asthmatic children, they scored higher on Wechsler perceptual motor subtests than on the purely verbal. As in previous studies with adults who had psychosomatic symptoms involving the body exterior, when the Rorschach inkblot test was scored for body image measures the arthritic children had high scores on the barrier index (i.e. a high number of responses involving objects with well-defined boundaries), their scores significantly exceeding those of the asthmatic children. Half of the mothers were depressed and felt guilt about the child's illness while the others tended to deny its existence.

LAMBERT, C.N.,
HAMILTON, R.C.,
and PELLICORE,
R.J.
(1969)
*Journal of Bone
and Joint Surgery,*
51-A, 6, 1135–8.

The juvenile amputee program: its social and economic value: a follow-up study after the age of 21

Of 150 men and women, with congenital or acquired amputations, who had been fitted with prostheses before the age of 21, over half were married, a third had children of their own, 112 were employed and 28 were students. 94 per cent of those with lower-limb prostheses and 61.2 per cent of those with upper limb prostheses wore them all day. The authors consider the cost of fitting children with prostheses well-justified, even in economic terms alone. Subjects on whom the findings were based were those who responded to a questionnaire sent to 246 former patients at an amputee clinic.

GRAHAM, P. and
RUTTER, M.
(1970)
In: RUTTER, M.,
TIZARD, J., and
WHITMORE, K.
(Eds), *Education,
Health and
Behaviour.*
London:
Longman, pp.
309–327.

Psychiatric aspects of physical disorder

There was a slight excess of psychiatric disorders among 10- to 12-year-old physically handicapped children (all disorders not involving the brain) living on the Isle of Wight, compared with that among the general population (10.4 per cent for the handicapped children and 6.6 per cent for the general population). Rates were similar for asthmatic children and for children with all other physical disorders (excluding those with brain dysfunction). Most of the physically handicapped children showed no disorder. As with non-handicapped children there was no tendency for neurotic or antisocial disorders to predominate. There was no association between the severity of the physical disability and psychiatric disorder.

KOHLBERG, L.J.
and
ROTHENBERG,
M.B.
(1970)
*American Journal
of Diseases of
Children,* 119, 5,
449–51.

Comprehensive care following multiple, life-threatening injuries: treatment of an adolescent boy

Case study of an adolescent boy who sustained severe injuries and permanent disabilities (including amputation) as a result of an accident. The case is described as demonstrating the emotions – fear, anger, guilt and sadness – invariably felt by the child and his family when sudden accident or illness disrupts ordinary life. An approach by which the paediatrician can deal with these reactions, both to facilitate treatment and avoid future psychological problems, is discussed. This consists of encouraging verbalization of thoughts and feelings, by use of a 'third person technique' (i.e. 'people in your situation often have feelings of this kind') if necessary.

MYERS, B.A.,
FRIEDMAN, S.B.,
and WEINER, I.B.
(1970)
*American Journal
of Diseases of
Children,* 120, 3,
175–181.

Coping with chronic disability. Psychosocial observations of girls with scoliosis, treated with the Milwaukee brace

Sixteen out of a sample of 26 girls (aged 9 to 16 years) were able to adjust well to the wearing of a Milwaukee brace for the treatment of scoliosis. Nine had serious problems in wearing the brace. The sample was biased, six girls being referred to the study particularly because of behaviour problems, while the others were randomly selected from the scoliosis patients seen at an orthopaedic clinic. Factors which aided adjustment were understanding of scoliosis and the reason for bracing, a conscious decision to wear the brace, an optimistic view of the outcome, support of the family and regular visits to the clinic. No significant relationship was found between the girls' adjustment to the brace and distorted body imagery as indicated by projective tests.

REITE, M.,
DAVIS,
K., SOLOMONS,
C.,
and OTT, J.
(1972)
*American Journal
of Psychiatry,* 128,
12, 1540–6.

Osteogenesis imperfecta: psychological function

Twelve cases of this rare disorder are described. Intelligence was normal, and interviews suggested that the children were well-adjusted. The authors speculate whether the metabolic energy disturbance associated with the disease might affect mood in a benign manner.

ADLER, S.N.M.
(1973)
*Dissertation
Abstracts
International,* 34,
3-B, 1266–7.

The stigma of handicap and its unlearning: a social perspective on children with muscle disease and their families

Children with physical handicaps have been found to be low in self-esteem; the study examined whether this could be improved. Home visits were made to the families of 25 children (22 boys, three girls) with various forms of muscular dystrophy, and the emotional climate of the family and the adjustment of the children observed. Many families were isolated and withdrawn from the sick child, prematurely grieving. The children all attended a one-week camp for children with chronic muscle disease, and for half of them special efforts were made to foster their talents and to express social approval. The other half acted as control group. Afterwards both groups of children were compared on projective drawings and sociogram scores. The experimental group, but not the controls, showed a significant increase in maturity and self-esteem on these tests. This result suggests that there could be great benefit in an early intervention programme for these children, together with self-help groups for the families, and attempts to re-educate public attitudes.

BENGTSSON, G.,
FÄLLSTRÖM, K.,
JANSSON, B., and
NACHEMSON, A.
(1974)
*Acta Psychiatrica
Scandinavica*, 50,
50–9.

A psychological and psychiatric investigation of the adjustment of female scoliosis

A study of the emotional adjustment of 26 women with idiopathic scoliosis. The deformity was appreciable in all cases. Fifteen of the 26 were married, and half worked full-time. Patients all underwent an extensive examination consisting of a structured interview, a general discussion, a projective test (Rorschach), the Bender test and an intelligence test. The degree of psychological handicap was assessed on a four-point scale. Two case histories are given.

Intelligence was normal or above normal. At the psychiatric examination, nine women were found to be under some treatment; but more than nine were considered to have a disturbance due to their disability. Socially, nearly half were considered to be well-adjusted; but in terms of personal adjustment only five were considered well-adjusted to their disability. The results suggest that the patients had developed a good social facade, but that most were depressed and insecure about the deformity, particularly if it was severe.

MCANARNEY,
E.R., PLESS, B.,
SATTERWHITE,
B.,
and FRIEDMAN,
S.B.
(1974)
Pediatrics, 53,
523–8.

Psychological problems of children with chronic juvenile arthritis

The adjustment of 42 children in New York with chronic arthritis was compared with a matched group of normal children. The arthritic children were sorted into three groups: non-disabled, mildly disabled, and moderately to severely disabled. Parents and teachers then filled in questionnaires about the children's adjustment, and the children themselves were given seven tests assessing intelligence, personality and adjustment.

Emotional health was judged to be 'excellent' by only 36 per cent of the arthritic children compared to 60 per cent of the controls. Twice as many of the arthritic children as of the controls had been referred to a school psychologist, and nearly three times as many had low achievement scores in spite of the fact that the intellectual ability of the two groups was similar. On the personality tests, more children with arthritis assessed themselves as 'different' or 'inferior'.

When the groups with varying degrees of disablement were compared, however, it was found that the group with the least disablement had the most psychological problems. The authors suggest that the arthritics without physical disablement received 'mixed messages' about their health and future and were thus under more stress than visibly handicapped children. Support for arthritic children and their families should be an integral part of out-patient services.

PLESS, I.B. and
PINKERTON, P.
(1975)
London: Henry
Kimpton.

Chronic Childhood Disorder

An overall survey of the emotional adjustment of the child with a chronically disabling disorder, assessing research and drawing conclusions from it. The concept of adjustment is discussed and the measures used to assess it are evaluated. The evidence for maladjustment in children with handicaps of many kinds is reviewed, and therapeutic intervention through the family, school and hospital delineated. Thirty pages of references are included.

CLAYSON, D.C.
and LEVINE, D.B.
(1976)
*Clinical
Orthopedics*, 116,
99–102.

Adolescent scoliosis patients: personality patterns and effects of corrective surgery

A group of 29 boys and 55 girls aged 12 to 20 with idiopathic scoliosis were given tests of personality before and after surgery. It appeared that the younger patients were less affected psychologically by their disability than the older ones. The boys showed comparatively better general personality integration than the girls, but were more disturbed in their psychosexual development. The girls were more affected by the operation than the boys. Boys depended on a feeling of self-acceptance, girls more on the acceptance of others, and post-operative care should take account of these differences. The earlier surgical correction can take place the better.

POPE-GRATTAN,
M.M., BURNETT,
C.N., and WOLFE,
C.V.
(1976)
Physical Therapy,
56, 168–76.

Human figure drawings by children with Duchenne's muscular dystrophy

Forty-three boys aged 4½ to 15 with muscular dystrophy were asked to 'draw a person'. The drawings were analysed systematically using 11 emotional indicators, and four personality traits were discovered to be common – physical inadequacy, immaturity, body anxiety and insecurity.

VOLPE, R.
(1976)
*Journal of Special
Education*, 10, 4,
371–81.

Orthopedic disability, restriction, and role-taking activity

Several hypotheses were examined: that disabled children would tend to take the role of patient and non-disabled children that of agent; that disabled children would be retarded in the achievement of 'concrete operations' (Piaget's definition of the intellectual stage reached by school-age children); and that disabled children would show a significantly lower level of role-taking than normal children. The hypotheses were tested by means of a battery of tests completed by 40 children with orthopaedic handicaps attending a hospital school in Canada, aged six to 12, and 40 matched non-disabled children. The tests included Piaget's conservation and classification tasks, a projective test assessing ability to take on roles shown in pictures, and two questionnaires assessing passivity and activity.

Results showed that the hypotheses were confirmed to some degree, the orthopaedically handicapped children tending to take a passive role, being slightly (though not significantly) more backward in carrying out the Piagetian tasks, and less active in role-taking on the picture tests. There was a tendency for the older handicapped children's scores to be closer to those of the control group, suggesting that there is increasing autonomy with age.

Fox, A.M.
(1977)
British Journal of Hospital Medicine, 17, 479–90.

Psychological problems of physically handicapped children

A detailed article on the general problems of the physically handicapped child, with the aim of teaching doctors how to approach both children and parents sensitively. The child knows he is 'different', and he may miss out on many of the normal accompaniments of growing up. The parents, rather than be made to feel incompetent in the face of professionals, should be encouraged to have confidence and impart it to the child, and in particular not to overprotect him. Information about the condition should be made available and comprehensible, and support should be available at crisis points.

Rimon, R.,
Belmaker, R.H.
and Ebstein, R.
(1977)
Scandinavian Journal of Rheumatology, 6, 1–10.

Psychosomatic aspects of juvenile rheumatoid arthritis

Previous studies have found a relationship between rheumatoid arthritis and emotional factors, and the purpose of the investigation was to pursue this. The subjects were 54 children with the disease admitted to hospital in Finland (16 boys, 30 girls). As well as the patients, 43 mothers, 20 fathers and 14 siblings were studied. Psychiatric profiles of the children were compiled by a psychiatrist, a psychologist, doctors and nurses; relatives were interviewed.

39 per cent of the children had previously suffered from an emotional disturbance, usually depressive. During the study 31 per cent were observed to have manifest psychopathology. Over half the children revealed a personality profile marked by shyness, unresponsiveness, passivity and inability to express emotion, traits which have been associated with rheumatoid arthritis in adults. Relationships with fathers were more often

disturbed than relationships with mothers (48 per cent and 33 per cent). In 37 per cent of the children a correlation between emotionally important conflict and the onset of the illness was observed. In the 63 per cent for whom there was no such correlation, the incidence of rheumatoid relatives was greater than in the former group.

It is concluded that there may be two categories: patients with a hereditary predisposition to the illness in whom the disease is less influenced by environmental changes, and patients with less hereditary predisposition in whom the onset of the disease is associated with psychodynamic conflict situations.

SCHATZINGER, L.A.H., NASH, C.L., DROTAR, D.D., and HALL, T.W. (1977) *Clinical Orthopedics*, 125, 145–50.

Emotional adjustment in scoliosis

The treatment of idiopathic scoliosis in adolescents with braces or surgery can cause emotional reactions. The study assessed personality and performance in 31 scoliosis patients in Ohio before and after treatment, and 92 cases were reviewed from case records. A battery of tests of personality, behaviour problems, intelligence and school achievement was administered to the sample of 31. All were found to be of average or good intelligence and were up to standard in their schoolwork. When the 92 cases were examined, only 12 per cent had no behavioural reactions to the use of the Milwaukee brace and 37 per cent to surgery. Those who already had problems had the greatest difficulty in coping with the scoliosis treatment.

HARPER, D.C. and RICHMAN, L.C. (1978) *Journal of Clinical Psychology*, 34, 636–42.

Personality profiles of physically impaired adolescents

Two groups of adolescents in Iowa with different disabilities (cleft palate and orthopaedic handicaps) were compared for their scores on the Minnesota Multiphasic Personality Inventory. In the orthopaedic group there were 28 boys and 18 girls, with a mean IQ of 96; their handicaps were varied, and ranged from moderate to severe. The cleft lip and palate group consisted of 30 boys and 22 girls with similar IQs. The results suggested different types of adjustment pattern; the cleft palate group's scores suggested difficulties in interpersonal relationships, while the orthopaedic group showed impulsivity in interpersonal relationships, and sensitivity about identity. The cleft palate group also displayed greater concern and ruminative doubt, while the orthopaedically handicapped showed a tendency to isolation and passivity. The findings support the belief that different types of disability produce different personality types in adolescents.

HENOCH, M.J.,
BATSON, J.W. and
BAUM, J.
(1978)
*Arthritis and
Rheumatism*, 21,
229–33.

Psychosocial factors in juvenile rheumatoid arthritis

Records of all children with juvenile rheumatoid arthritis over 16 years at a hospital in New York were surveyed, and 88 cases (67 girls, 21 boys) found willing to be studied. Data from a child population study were used as a comparison. There were no racial or socioeconomic biases among the arthritis patients. The female/male ratio was representative of the distribution of the disease. Children whose parents were single due to death or divorce comprised 28 per cent of the arthritis group compared to 11 per cent of the comparison group; adoption was three times as common in the arthritis group as in the comparison group. About half the deaths, divorces and adoptions took place within the two years before the onset of the disease. Half of the families reported some history of arthritis, but many of the reports were vague. The authors conclude that there seems to be a strong correlation between stress and the onset of juvenile rheumatoid arthritis.

SIEGEL, I.M. and
KORNFELD, M.S.
(1980)
Physical Therapy,
60, 293–8.

Kinetic family drawing test for evaluating families having children with muscular dystrophy

An exploratory study of the use of a drawing test to learn about the feelings and conflicts of boys and their families with muscular dystrophy. Ten boys with muscular dystrophy and ten of their siblings were asked to draw all members of the family doing something. The children's drawings were discussed in relation to the problems expressed in them. The siblings of the disabled children showed some ambivalence and anger. Identification with fathers was weak. The boys with muscular dystrophy showed dependence on the mother. It is suggested that the drawing test is a useful tool in assessing and helping these patients.

WILKINSON, V.A.
(1981)
*International
Rehabilitation
Medicine*, 3,
11–17.

Juvenile chronic arthritis in adolescence: facing the reality

The study was based on 17 in-patients with juvenile chronic arthritis and nine out-patients (a total of eight boys and 18 girls). Ages ranged from 12 to 19. Each patient was seen for a semi-structured psychiatric interview, and parents were also interviewed. Patients' records were reviewed and medical and nursing staff, teachers and social workers were interviewed.

The patients were found to be very socially isolated, even those who were out-patients. Most of the girls expressed an interest in meeting the opposite sex, but only two of the eight boys did. A large proportion of these adolescents were small for their age, due to taking corticosteroids, and over half were limited in mobility; these factors were linked with depression. The patients also expressed anxiety about their mobility and about plans for the future; pain was not a main source of concern. Nearly all subjects expressed a preference for going to an ordinary school and wanted more friends among the able-bodied. Plans for the future were more realistic among the out-patients than among the in-patients.

In eight families out of the 26 there were deaths and divorces and seven of the broken families had suffered additional stresses. There was a marked tendency for depressive symptoms to be associated with broken families. Eleven of the mothers had sought help for depression, but there appeared to be no correlation between depression in mothers and in their children. It was considered that 19 of the 26 families were supportive to the child. Nine in-patients and two out-patients had been referred for psychiatric assessment for depression and anxiety, and one girl had attempted suicide. More girls than boys had psychiatric referrals. Clearly these young people are isolated, anxious about sexual problems, and depressed about their future, though the out-patient group was less handicapped in these ways than the in-patients. Their psychiatric problems should be taken seriously rather than dismissed as part of the disease.

ANDERSON, F.J. (1982) *Issues in Mental Health Nursing,* 4, 4, 257–74.

Self-concept and coping in adolescents with a physical disability

The relationship between self-concept and coping with a physical disability is complex. When 59 adolescent girls with scoliosis were examined on a 'self-concept scale', they were found to have no more negative feelings about themselves than would a representative sample of non-disabled girls. A surgeon and an orthopaedic clinic nurse, asked to rate the girls' self-concept, disagreed both with each other and with the girls' self-ratings and assessments of coping style. It may be unhelpful for patients if health care professionals are not in touch with what patients themselves are thinking.

BEALES, J.G.,
LENNOX HOLT,
P.J., KEEN, J.H.,
and MELLOR,
V.P.
(1983)
*Annals of the
Rheumatic
Diseases*, 42,
481–6.

Children with juvenile chronic arthritis: their beliefs about their illness and therapy

In order to ascertain their beliefs about their illness, 75 young patients with juvenile chronic arthritis in Manchester (ages 7 to 17) were asked about what they believed the illness to be and what their therapy was for. Each also drew a picture of what the joints looked like and was asked what he felt about his picture.

A broad difference was observed between the younger and the older patients' attitudes. Younger children saw the disease in terms of their symptoms, and had only vague ideas of physiology ('something is gluing my bones together'). Most of the patients over 12 perceived arthritis as a state of internal pathology, though they too were unable to give a correct account of the physiology of arthritis and saw it in exaggerated and simplified terms. The younger children's drawings were naive; the older ones had more ability to show haemorrhaging and internal damage. The older children, but not the younger, tended to say that they were upset or repelled by the damage they had depicted. The younger group disliked and misunderstood their splints, medications and injections, the older group accepted that there was a beneficial connection with the illness. It might be wise to give the children more information about their condition, phrased in terms suited to their age.

BEALES, J.G.,
KEEN, J.H. and
LENNOX HOLT,
P.J.
(1983)
*Journal of
Rheumatology*,
10, 61–5.

The child's perception of the disease and the experience of pain in juvenile chronic arthritis

Interviews conducted among 39 young patients with juvenile chronic arthritis supported the hypothesis that the meaning which the child attributes to sensations in the joints influences the extent to which those sensations constitute pain. Joint sensation was assessed by presenting to the child a list of items (burning, aching) and asking him to describe what the sensations meant to him. He then assessed the extent of pain on a scale from 'not at all nasty' to 'the worst pain you can imagine'. All the children reported aching and other sensations, but the younger children did not associate these with unpleasant ideas. To the older child, however, the sensations were more distressing because they reminded them of their disability ('it makes me sad'). They visualized unpleasant conditions underneath the skin. 58 per cent of the children over 12 scored above midpoint on the scale of pain, while only 20 per cent of the younger children did. It is concluded that 'pain' means something different and worse to the child as he grows older.

SHINDI, J.
(1983)
*International
Journal of Social
Psychiatry*, 29, 4,
292–8.

Emotional adjustment of physically handicapped children: a comparison of children with congenital and acquired orthopaedic disabilities

A comparison was made between 20 children with congenital orthopaedic handicaps and 20 with acquired ones. All the children filled in three questionnaires assessing various attitudes. The congenital group's scores showed that they had more guilt than the other group; while the group with acquired handicaps showed more sense of isolation and bitterness. In general the latter group seemed to be more emotionally maladjusted. Girls showed more maladjustment than boys.

The author suggests that the children with congenital disabilities may have absorbed from parents a sense that to be born with a handicap was some sort of punishment, while the other group knew specifically what to blame for their disability. On the other hand, the group with acquired disabilities had less support from the family and also had the problem of adjusting to a changed life.

STANDEN, P.J.
(1983)
*Psychological
Medicine*, 13, 4,
847–54.

The long-term psychological adjustment of children treated for congenital dislocation of the hip

In order to determine whether early hospitalization is detrimental to children's mental health, a group of 81 children with congenital dislocation of the hip (nearly all girls) were compared with three other matched groups. Children with this disability have to spend some months in hospital at an early age, experiencing operations and periods of immobilization. The three comparison groups were (i) 44 children who had had a hospital admission of less than a week before the age of five; (ii) 26 children who had had two or more admissions, one before five; (iii) 51 children with no experience of hospital admission. Psychological adjustment was measured by means of Rutter's questionnaires for parents and teachers. Both the parental and the teachers' questionnaires selected more children with signs of maladjustment in the hip dislocation group. There was a suggestion, though, that the maladjustment was concentrated among the younger children, implying that perhaps they may grow out of it.

GRATZ, R. and
PAPALIA-FINLAY,
D.
(1984)
*Journal of
Adolescent Health
Care,* 5, 237–42.

Psychosocial adaptation to wearing the Milwaukee brace

The psychological and social effects of wearing a brace for
scoliosis were examined in interviews and questionnaires with 16
mothers and daughters. Results suggested that after the initial
shock of learning about the condition, the brace was quite well
accepted. Problems mentioned included buying clothes,
limitation of movement, and the fear of unkind comments.
Participation in sports and hobbies was not seriously affected.

SECTION III
Family Adjustment

In this book and in its companion volumes, the problems of bringing up a handicapped child, whatever the handicap, are reported in very similar fashion. There is the question of finding out about the disability, either at birth if it is obvious or later if it is not. In the former case parents report shock, distress and incredulity, gradually changing in most cases to acceptance of the position and love for the child (Drotar *et al.*, 1975; Buchanan *et al.*, 1979; McKeever, 1981). When a diagnosis has had to be obtained later, many parents have reported a long time of waiting before one was definitely offered – two-and-a-half years in the case of the sample studied by Firth (1983). Many parents in his sample felt they had not been sensitively told, nor given enough information. As the child grows up, it would seem that in particular the parents of muscular dystrophy children could benefit from extra support and counselling (Buchanan *et al.*, 1979; Kornfeld and Siegel, 1979).

The practical side of caring for a handicapped child is described by Carnegie United Kingdom Trust (1964) and Baldwin (1977). Orthopaedic handicaps in particular may involve a wheelchair life and all that it entails (Russell, 1984 (see Section V)). It is clear that parents often have problems with adapting their houses, installing mobility aids, and meeting extra costs. Few studies have expressed satisfaction with the kind of practical and emotional support available for families where there is a child with any kind of handicap.

CARNEGIE
UNITED
KINGDOM TRUST
(1964)
Edinburgh: J. and
A. Constable.
(Part I,
Appendices G and
H; Part II,
Chapters 4 and 5;
Part III, Chapter
6.)

Handicapped Children and their Families

Studies of children with orthopaedic handicaps and their families were made as part of a larger survey of the needs of all types of handicapped children. Research was carried out in three areas, Glasgow, Sheffield and Shropshire. A mass of data on the practical problems involved in the care of physically handicapped children was accumulated. Parental attitudes were found to be a crucial factor in the child's adjustment.

DOW, T.E.
(1965)
*Psychological
Reports*, 17, 1,
39–62.

Social class and reaction to physical disability

The main purpose of this study was to investigate the hypothesis that reaction to disability would be more severe in lower-class families, due to their dependence on physical means to obtain economic success. Fifty-eight New Jersey families with a child hospitalized for an orthopaedic or medical condition were interviewed and administered questionnaires. Contrary to the hypothesis, parental attitudes to disability were uniformly optimistic, regardless of social class. In their actual behaviour, family reaction to the medical diagnosis was related to family size, not social class. Small families reacted in an extreme manner, normal family life being completely disrupted. Large families reacted in a balanced manner, the parents adopting the least disruptive course. While the parents generally de-emphasized the importance of physique, this was not so uniformly true for the children. Emphasis on physique was related to the child's prospects of recovery.

DROTAR, D.,
BASKIEWICZ, A.,
IRVIN, N.,
KENNELL, J., and
KLAUS, M.
(1975)
Pediatrics, 56, 5,
710–17.

The adaptation of parents to the birth of an infant with a congenital malformation: a hypothetical model

Interviews were held with parents of 20 children with a range of common congenital malformations hospitalized in Ohio. Timing of the interviews ranged from within a few days of birth to as long as five years later, 65 per cent being in the first year. Parents were asked a series of open-ended questions to determine their emotional reactions and perception of the child's handicap.

A number of common themes emerged, and five stages of reaction were delineated. Shock: the initial response was overwhelming shock. All but two parents reported a sense of abrupt disruption of normality. Denial: many tried to escape or deny the situation. Sadness, anger, anxiety: this accompanied and followed denial. Seven families reported feeling anger towards themselves, the baby, or hospital staff and others. Eleven described intense feelings of anxiety. Five spontaneously spoke of fears that the baby might die and this seemed related to hesitance seen in almost all the mothers regarding their attachment to the child. Adaptation: ten reported a gradual lessening in anxiety and confidence in their ability to care for the child. Many mothers emphasized the child's normal qualities, and this appeared to reflect positive adaptation rather than denial of the disability. Reorganization: a complex time in which a more rewarding level of interaction with the child was described. Some parents continued to search for causes of the disability, while three seemed content that it had 'just happened'. Positive long-term acceptance involved parents' mutual support of one another, seven couples reporting that they had relied closely on one another, and six that the experience had brought them closer together. Asynchronous parental reactions often resulted in temporary emotional separation and may be a significant factor in separations following major family crises.

Marked loneliness and anxieties immediately after the birth were common, and the study suggests that generally the child should be brought to the parents as soon as possible after birth and the problems discussed, emphasizing the infant's normal attributes. Paediatric advice, support and counselling during the first year of the baby's life will be crucial to maximizing the child's development and the adjustment of the family.

BALDWIN, S.
(1977)
The Disability
Alliance.

Disabled Children – Counting the Costs

In order to get an idea of the cost of bringing up a handicapped child, interviews were carried out with parents of 303 severely handicapped children in Britain. The commonest cause of reduced income was the inability of the child's mother to take paid work outside the home. The father's work was often also affected; nearly a quarter said they had had to give up overtime or to turn down a job at a distance from home. Altogether, 47 per cent of the sample said that the family income had gone down as a result of the handicapped child's special needs.

Secondly, there were extra expenses: heating, house adaptations (a third of the families had made adaptations and half of these had borne the full cost), repairing damage caused by the child, installing mobility aids (over a third had paid for these themselves). Transport to hospital was not always provided by ambulance, and the cost of visiting a child in hospital or in a residential school had to be paid for. The mobility allowance available to certain groups of handicapped children was not adequate.

Another important cause of extra expenditure was incontinence – aids such as nappies and creams had to be bought, extra washing to be done, and there was expenditure on clothes and bedding. Finally, clothes, shoes and bedding got extra wear in 85 per cent of the families and caused further expenditure, and some families had to spend extra money on food. In all, 90 per cent of the families quoted some extra costs, and the more severe the handicap the higher the cost. Further state benefits for these families are essential.

BUCHANAN,
D.C.,
LaBARBERA,
C.J.,
ROELOFS, R., and
OLSON, W.
(1979)
*General Hospital
Psychiatry*, 1,
262–9.

Reactions of families to children with Duchenne muscular dystrophy

Twenty-five families were interviewed to examine their adjustment to having a child with Duchenne muscular dystrophy. The children were aged 4 to 14. 64 per cent of the families had no known family history of the disease, while seven families (28 per cent) had a known history (in two families it was impossible to ascertain the history because the mother had left). Response to the diagnosis was particularly traumatic for those with no known family history; some parents had been put on psychiatric drugs, one mother attempted suicide, and two mothers abandoned the family. Divorce (28 per cent) was not higher than the national average, but a further quarter of the couples were having serious marital problems which often seemed to relate to the child's illness. Four of the families, however, felt that the child's birth had strengthened their marriages.

The majority of parents mentioned psychological problems rather than practical ones as their major difficulty. Twenty-one mothers said they would advise other carriers of the illness not to have children. Psychological problems included the unpredictable course of the illness, social stigma, and guilt in the mother about genetic transmission. Many parents coped only by partly denying the disease or by over-protecting the child. Other family members were also affected; some siblings seemed to be disturbed, and grandparents, though supportive, sometimes interfered or spoiled the affected child. Some of the children themselves showed signs of emotional disturbance, a feeling that their 'weak muscles' were their own fault, and a need to know more about the disease. Over half the children were in private or special schools, and parents were often dissatisfied with their education. The most helpful things enabling the parents to cope were an ability to communicate, a concentration on the present, some kind of outside interest or recreation, and support from people outside the nuclear family.

KORNFELD, M.S.
and SIEGEL, I.M.
(1979)
*Health and Social
Work,* 4, 3,
99–118.

Parental group therapy in the management of a fatal childhood disease

A discussion of the issues faced in a therapy group for parents of boys with muscular dystrophy. Among other points, parents realized that they focused more on the child's physical problems than his psychological ones, that they indulged the disabled too much and sometimes took out their feelings on non-handicapped siblings, and that they found it hard to face up to the question of sexuality in their sons. Sharing problems in a group helped them to accept the disease and handle these problems.

McKEEVER, P.T.
(1981)
*Maternal Child
Nursing Journal,*
6, 124–8.

Fathering the chronically ill child

Ten fathers of children with a variety of disablements were interviewed to determine their feelings about their role. All found it difficult to talk about their feelings, but none withdrew from the study. Five main areas of concern were discussed.

Communication with health professionals: fathers had had considerably less contact with health professionals than their wives. None felt they had been really prepared for the child's progress. Effects of the handicap: first reactions had been of shock and disbelief. Fathers restricted their lives a good deal to stay and help the family. Marriages were strengthened and weakened by the situation in about equal proportions. Involvement with the handicapped child: fathers in general were deeply involved, in contrast to the findings of some other research. They felt that they and not the doctor should explain the child's condition to him. Coping mechanisms: the men tended to deny the severity of the handicap to cope with their feelings. In general they did not confide much in outsiders about the problem. Main concerns: fathers worried about the day-to-day unpredictability of the child's condition, but in particular worried about the future and the adult life ahead of their child. Many worried about their wives' health, describing depression, fatigue and anxiety.

In general the fathers interviewed seemed to be coping courageously. Their needs should be recognized as well as those of their wives. Caretakers to facilitate outings and holidays for these families are urgently needed. The study should be replicated with a larger sample, comparing the responses of mothers, fathers and siblings.

FIRTH, M.A.
(1983)
*British Medical
Journal*, 286,
700–1.

Diagnosis of Duchenne muscular dystrophy: experiences of parents of sufferers

Fifty-three families where there was a son with Duchenne muscular dystrophy were interviewed about their experiences in obtaining a diagnosis of the disease. The average time between their becoming aware of symptoms and the final diagnosis was two-and-a-half-years. Many parents were given another diagnosis and then had to face a different and more devastating one. Only in 18 of the 53 families were both parents told together. Fifteen of them were not satisfied with the way they had been told; these families had had on average a longer time to wait before getting the correct diagnosis. Many parents complained of not being given enough information; it is difficult for this to be taken in at one interview, and arrangements should be made for further interviews. Parents should also be told as much as possible as early as possible, and should be told together in private.

SECTION IV
Educational Attainments

Orthopaedic handicaps form such a mixed group that there is no study attempting to assess the educational attainments of the group as a whole. The next best thing is Yule and Rutter's (1970) section of the Isle of Wight project that deals with children with physical disorders. Disabilities involving the brain were excluded, as were eczema and asthma, and the group remaining consisted of 43 children of whom 15 had orthopaedic handicaps. The average IQ was slightly below that of a control group, and there was a degree of reading backwardness; 16.7 per cent were reading at a level at least 28 months below that expected for their age and intelligence, as compared to 5.4 per cent in the control group.

Apart from this, there is a concentration of research on muscular dystrophy patients. The evidence is reviewed by Karagan (1979); some 40 studies are discussed and the overwhelming conclusion is that these children suffer from a slight degree of mental retardation which cannot be ascribed to anxiety or a socially limited life. A number of the studies are included here. The retardation is not progressive and has no association with the degree of physical handicap. There is evidence that verbal intelligence is more affected than the skills tested on the performance subscale (Marsh and Munsat, 1974; Karagan and Zellweger, 1978).

A few studies relating to educating the physically handicapped in ordinary schools are included here. Anderson (1973) studied a number of the physically handicapped being educated in primary and junior schools. The children who were handicapped in attainment and social mixing tended to be those with brain involvement rather than orthopaedic handicaps. Cope and Anderson (1977) then studied physically handicapped children in special units attached to ordinary schools, and came to the conclusion that the best units offered as good an education as the special schools, with the advantage of contact with non-handicapped peers. Hegarty *et al.* (1981, 1982) and Hodgson *et al.* (1984) have described in some detail how different schemes of integration are being carried out in schools across the country.

WORDEN, D.K.
and VIGNOS, P.J.
(1962)
Pediatrics, 29, 6,
968–77.

Intellectual function in childhood progressive muscular dystrophy

Thirty-eight patients with muscular dystrophy aged four to 17 years (mean age 11) had a mean IQ of 83, and mean educational quotients of 84 and 87 in arithmetic and reading respectively. There was no significant link with the severity of the physical disability, duration of the illness, or age, and therefore no evidence to suggest mental deterioration. Among the siblings of 27 patients, mean IQ was 110. Comparison was also made with a group of diabetics and a group of children having amyotonia congenita to determine whether chronic illness or locomotor restriction caused lowered intelligence; the mean scores of these two groups were 107 and 118. The mental as well as the physical handicap in muscular dystrophy must be realistically assessed.

DUBOWITZ, V.
(1965)
*Archives of
Disease in
Childhood,* 40,
296–301.

Intellectual impairment in muscular dystrophy

A careful study was made of 63 boys and two girls, aged three to 19, by three methods; a long-term assessment of intelligence based on observation, full intelligence tests administered to 27 of the sample, and detailed prospective case studies of three patients. The conclusions were that less than half the group could be considered to be within the normal range of intelligence and development. Lower intelligence was related to a positive family history. Reasons for the intellectual impairment are discussed.

DAGUE, P.
(1970)
*Revue de
Neuropsychiatrie
Infantile et
d'Hygiène Mentale
de l'Enfance,* 18,
319–45.

Mental levels in myopathy

108 boys with Duchenne-type muscular dystrophy, aged five to 15 years, had a mean IQ of 82.9. 40 per cent had an IQ below 80. The degree of intellectual retardation was not associated with age, stage of the disease, type of genetic transmission, serum enzyme level or disturbance in EEG. Siblings of the subjects generally had normal intelligence. Possible explanations for the findings are discussed.

DAGUE, P. and
TEMBOURY, M.
(1970)
*Revue de
Neuropsychiatrie
Infantile et
d'Hygiène Mentale
de L'Enfance,* 18,
347–76.

Study of some aspects of the mental activity and the behaviour at school of children with myopathy

Perception and memory and aspects of school behaviour (attention, comprehension, memory, effort, work rhythm, discipline, attitude to schoolwork and manual or artistic aptitude) were studied in children with muscular dystrophy and control groups of normal children and children with physical disabilities but no motor handicaps. The children with muscular dystrophy were inferior to the other groups on all aspects.

YULE, W. and
RUTTER, M.
(1970)
In: RUTTER, M.,
TIZARD, J. and
WHITMORE, K.
(Eds) *Education,
Health and
Behaviour,*
London:
Longman, pp.
297–308.

Educational aspects of physical disorder

As part of a large-scale survey of handicapping conditions in children, aged 10 to 12 years, living on the Isle of Wight, those with physical disorders were identified (see also Graham and Rutter (1970) in Section II on 'Emotional and social adjustment'). Excluding those whose physical disorders involved the brain and those with asthma or eczema, there were 43 children with a wide variety of physical disabilities, including 15 with orthopaedic handicaps. The majority of these children were attending ordinary schools. The average IQ of the group was slightly below that of the Isle of Wight control group (on the shortened version of the Wechsler Intelligence Scale for Children). This group of children also showed reading backwardness (on the Neale Analysis of Reading Ability Test). 16.7 per cent were reading at a level at least 28 months below that expected on the basis of their age and IQ, compared with 5.4 per cent in the control group. A strong relationship was found between reading retardation and absence from school.

FAIR, D.T. and
BIRCH, J.W.
(1971)
*Exceptional
Children,* 38, 4,
335–6.

Effect of rest on test scores of physically handicapped and non-handicapped children

Physically handicapped children had better scores on the second part of a section of the Advanced Stanford Achievement test when they were allowed a rest between the parts, although a rest made no difference to non-handicapped children of comparable age, IQ and grade level. It is concluded that physically handicapped children should be given rest periods when taking standardized tests.

MARSH, G.G.
(1972)
*Perceptual and
Motor Skills,* 35,
504–6.

Impaired visual-motor ability of children with Duchenne muscular dystrophy

Twenty-one boys aged six to 13 with muscular dystrophy, from a California clinic, completed the Bender-Gestalt test which assesses visual-motor ability. They also took the WISC intelligence tests; mean scores were 85 for Verbal IQ and 93.3 for Performance IQ (full score 87.9). The Bender-Gestalt drawings were compared to drawings typical for the child's age. Of 21, 14 showed mild to severe visual-motor impairment, a proportion much higher than would be expected in a normal population. Poor scores on the Bender test were related to lower scores on the intelligence tests.

ANDERSON, E.M.
(1973)
London:
Methuen.

The Disabled Schoolchild

A study of the integration of physically handicapped children into primary schools. Seventy-four juniors, with matched non-handicapped control children, were studied, and also a group of 25 from infant schools. The sample was drawn from seven local education authorities in town and country.

School placement: Nearly half the parents of the handicapped children reported dissatisfaction with initial procedures for school placement; about 13 per cent of the juniors had been refused at first by schools, and many parents had had to put up a fight to get placement in an ordinary school. The majority would have disliked placement in a special school.

Social adjustment: This was assessed for all children by a sociometric test, and the handicapped children proved to be less popular than their able-bodied controls. According to parents' reports, about half the handicapped children were teased, but teachers only reported teasing in a much smaller number. The teasing was confined to urban schools.

Behaviour disorders: All children were assessed by the Rutter questionnaires; no difference was found between the handicapped group and the control group (but both groups had higher scores than the children in Rutter's Isle of Wight study – see p.18). Children with neurological abnormalities, such as the cerebral palsied, had a higher rate of behaviour disorder than the other handicapped children. For all children, antisocial behaviour disorder was much commoner than neurotic disorder.

Social competence: The handicapped children had lower scores than the non-handicapped children; neurological abnormality, severer handicap and lower intelligence were associated with lower scores.

Intelligence: There was no significant difference between the control group and the children without neurological abnormality, but the group with neurological abnormality had lower scores. The same applied to arithmetic and reading scores.

The author concludes with a discussion of how to integrate physically handicapped children into ordinary schools, and a comparison with school integration in Scandinavia.

MARSH, G.G. and
MUNSAT, T.L.
(1974)
Archives of
Disease in
Childhood, 49,
118–22.

Evidence for early impairment of verbal intelligence in Duchenne muscular dystrophy

A sample of 34 dystrophic boys aged five to 15 were given the full-scale WISC intelligence test. The younger, mildly disabled boys had a mean IQ of 90.37 and the older group of 87.44. When verbal subscores and performance subscores were compared, the less disabled group had a verbal IQ 12 points lower than their performance IQ. The older group had a similarly low verbal IQ, but their performance score was lower, probably due to increased muscle weakness. The authors conclude that in muscular dystrophy there is an early and non-progressive impairment of verbal intelligence, that there is some organic brain damage, tending to be verbal in nature, which is genetically determined and shows itself early. Teachers should not assume, however, that intelligence deteriorates as muscular weakness progresses.

COPE, C. and
ANDERSON, E.
(1977)
University of
London Institute
of Education.

Special Units in Ordinary Schools

A survey of special classes or units for physically handicapped children attached to primary and secondary schools in England and Wales. It was carried out by letter, visits and by a comparison of 55 children at special units with 55 in special schools. The children, matched for severity of handicap, were discussed with teachers and parents and were individually tested.

The children in the units were generally equal in basic educational attainments to those in special schools. Facilities such as ancillary helpers and material resources, however, were less good in the units than in the special schools, except in the two purpose-built units. At the secondary level in particular there was a shortage of physiotherapy and of arrangements for PE classes. Children in special units and special schools expressed themselves as equally happy in their school lives. A higher proportion of special school than of unit children were not chosen as friends by other children. On a scale of social competence, the unit children had a significantly higher self-direction score than the other group. On assessments of adjustment and behaviour, both groups were similar. At the secondary level, handicapped children did not appear to be segregated or subjected to teasing.

The degree of classroom integration varied from school to school, the main barrier being limited ability in the handicapped pupil. At the secondary level there was more flexibility and more mixing. At both primary and secondary level, social integration was easier to achieve than academic integration. In general, there was a fair amount of integration, which was beneficial to the handicapped child; but more could have been achieved if it had been a major goal for the school. The best units offered as good an education as the special schools, together with the benefit of contact with non-handicapped peers.

The authors recommend a shift in policy towards more special provision within the ordinary school, and add 46 detailed recommendations about implementation.

FLOREK, M. and
KAROLAK, S.
(1977)
*European Journal
of Pediatrics*, 126,
275–82.

Intelligence level of patients with Duchenne type of progressive muscular dystrophy

It has been established that muscular dystrophy patients have slightly lowered average intelligence levels. Various explanations have been proposed: socioeconomic deprivation, motor restriction, emotional disturbance, and causes related either directly or at a secondary level to the disease itself. To investigate this, four groups of boys in Poland aged four to 15 were compared: (i) 58 patients without complicating factors; (ii) 23 patients with a poor perinatal history; (iii) 36 patients from poor environments, either institutions or remote villages; (iv) 12 patients with both perinatal and environmental factors in their history. A comparative investigation was made of 27 children with Werding-Hoffman spinal muscular atrophy, a more severely limiting disease even than muscular dystrophy.

Average intelligence level was 79. Group (i) had an IQ of 85; group (ii) did not differ significantly from this. Group (iii) had a significantly lower intelligence level than the groups without adverse environmental factors. A comparison with the Werding-Hoffman group showed that this group had an average intelligence level of 98, significantly higher than that of the muscular dystrophy patients. EEG investigations of the muscular dystrophy group found only 17.2 per cent of records to be without pathological or borderline features.

It is concluded that there is a direct relation between muscular dystrophy and lowered intelligence level, although poor environmental conditions and increased immobility both depress the IQ score still further.

KARAGAN, N.J.
and ZELLWEGER,
H.U.
(1978)
*Developmental
Medicine and
Child Neurology,*
20, 4, 435–41.

Early verbal disability in children with Duchenne muscular dystrophy

An examination of the verbal/performance discrepancy in the IQ scores of muscular dystrophic children. The sample was confined to 53 boys aged five to 10, so that all the children would be ambulant and all the scores be on the same intelligence test, the WISC. When scores were examined, the mean verbal IQ was 80.66, 7.40 points lower than the mean performance IQ. When the scores were examined again two groups emerged, one with only lowered verbal ability and one with low scores on both verbal and performance scores. The results indicate a general, early verbal disability in muscular dystrophy patients, perhaps related to the direct physical influence of the disease on central nervous functioning. In some patients, non-verbal intellectual skills are impaired as well, which may be due to the same cause. Further study of brain–behaviour relationships in dystrophic patients is indicated.

KARAGAN, N.J.
(1979)
*Psychological
Bulletin,* 86, 2,
250–9.

Intellectual functioning in Duchenne muscular dystrophy: a review

A review of some 40 studies on the intelligence of boys with muscular dystrophy. The overwhelming conclusion is that they show some mental retardation when compared with the non-handicapped or those with other handicaps, and that it cannot be ascribed to limited social interaction. Verbal IQ is lowered more than performance IQ. The relation of this finding to the possible aetiology of the disease is discussed.

ALLSOP, J.
(1980)
*Journal of
Research and
Development in
Education,* 13, 4,
37–44.

Mainstreaming physically handicapped students

A practical discussion of the details of integrating physically handicapped children into ordinary classes. Headteachers should try to get to know the children before admission; and for the teachers, in-service training sessions can be held to learn about various disabilities. In the classroom, there must be adequate room for crutches and wheelchairs, and somewhere for children to rest. Practical adaptations to chairs and desks are suggested. The handicapped child should be subject to the same discipline as the other children, but schoolwork may need to be adapted or scaled down. The class can be helped to understand something about handicap before the child arrives. Factors influencing the decision that a child can be successfully integrated are discussed.

HEGARTY, S.
(1980)
Special Education,
7, 1, 8–10.

Integration – some questions to ask

As more children with special needs are being integrated into ordinary schools, a number of questions about their reception and education arise. The author identifies a number of relevant issues: introducing the children; staff requirements; curriculum adaptation; social interaction; transport and other practical arrangements; liaison with parents.

HEGARTY, S.,
POCKLINGTON, K.
and LUCAS, D.
(1981)
Windsor: NFER-
Nelson.

Educating Pupils with Special Needs in the Ordinary School

A three-year study of educational integration in 14 LEAs in this country. There were 17 integration programmes, ranging from nursery up to school-leaving age. Staff were interviewed at length.

Initiation: Procedures for starting an integration programme are discussed – talks with headteacher, preparation of school staff, telling the parents of children already in the school (not widely practised), preparation of the pupils themselves (also not very common). Things were frequently found to go wrong with preparation – handicapped pupils arriving before physical adaptations had been done, school staff not properly informed, initial support not maintained.

Staffing: The majority of the schools had special centres attached. Teachers staffing them varied widely in experience and background. Their duties included teaching the handicapped pupils, monitoring progress and integration, administrative work, giving information to ordinary staff, training, contacting parents, support teaching. Ancillaries were used in all the programmes studied, and their roles ranged from giving physical help to helping with schoolwork or physiotherapy. They were sometimes assigned to secondary schools, which could lead to difficulties with teachers. Of the ordinary teachers, only 36 out of 242 interviewed said they had a good knowledge of handicap; 43 said they had no knowledge at all. The great majority said that specialized knowledge of handicap was important in teaching children with special needs. Nearly 40 per cent said they had received insufficient information about the handicapped children they taught, often because of medical confidentiality.

Support from outside agencies such as educational psychologists and speech therapists was often insufficient. Asked about gains and losses from the integration programme, the main gain mentioned by teachers was the lack of social prejudice in the non-handicapped pupils. Losses included difficulties with timetabling and classroom allocation, discipline problems, and the question of incorporating the handicapped child into teaching geared to the majority. The roles of advisory teachers, educational psychologists, physiotherapists, doctors and speech therapists are discussed. Training: it appeared that many programmes are operating without appropriately trained staff, and there is much need for training. Pupils' needs were going unrecognized because of lack of awareness or competence on the part of staff.

The physical environment: Some of the needs to be taken into account are parking facilities, a level or ramped approach, wide doorways, lifts or internal ramps, suitable toilets, treatment room, fire escape routes, accessible play areas, meeting places and lunch rooms, staffroom for special centre, meeting room for parents. Costing issues are discussed in detail.

The curriculum: A number of the schools' adapted curricula are described. Factors influencing the allocation of handicapped pupils to various programmes are distinguished. Teachers indicated ways in which they modified their teaching approach – e.g. giving more individual attention, simplifying material. They reported many practical difficulties in teaching children with special needs: inability to give enough personal attention, uncertainty about the child's potential, discipline problems. Preparation for adult life: courses were given for school-leavers, both in relation to employment and to general life skills. Special attention was paid in many schools to keeping records of the handicapped pupils' progress.

Social interaction: This was easier for the younger handicapped children than the older. There were many examples of handicapped children only associating with the other handicapped. Positive steps need to be taken to improve social integration, but there was some ground for guarded optimism. In general, the handicapped pupils seemed more confident and mature than they would have been in special schools, but less so than the ordinary pupils. They made some progress in independence and lost some of their over-sensitivity. There was, however, a minority who were aggressive, bizarre or sexually precocious. Ordinary pupils, in general, accepted them, though not necessarily as fully-fledged members of the community. Teachers' attitudes were very positive; and parents without exception wanted ordinary schooling for the handicapped child. The main conclusion drawn from the study is that integrated education *is* possible, and to a far greater extent than is currently the practice.

LEIBOWITZ, D.
and DUBOWITZ,
V.
(1981)
*Developmental
Medicine and
Child Neurology,*
23, 5, 577–90.

Intellect and behaviour in Duchenne muscular dystrophy

The study attempts to answer the following questions: what is the overall level of intellectual functioning of dystrophic children? has it any particular pattern? how well can the children read? what are their behaviour patterns according to parents and teachers? what is the effect of age and disability? how do the children compare with normal children and other handicapped children? Subjects were 57 boys in London aged three to 13. They were given an intelligence test, a 'draw-a-man' test, a Bender copying test, a reading test, and parents and teachers were given behaviour questionnaires.

On the intelligence test, verbal scores were significantly lower than the performance scores. On the drawing test, scores were rather poor, showing immaturity, and on the copying test scores were below average. Reading, overall, was backward. On all these tests there was a proportion of children who scored at average level. On the behaviour questionnaire (teachers), 19 of 52 boys tested had scores suggesting maladjustment; this was true of more of the younger than the older boys. On similar questionnaires (parents), 18 out of 55 tested showed signs of maladjustment. This is a higher rate than has been found among physically handicapped children without cerebral involvement.

It is likely that muscular dystrophy is a disease affecting the central nervous system and thus linked with intelligence test and reading test results; the emotional disturbance, however, could be directly connected with the tragic implications of the disease. It is important for all those concerned with muscular dystrophic children to know that they are at risk of intellectual impairment, associated with educational retardation and emotional disturbance. For the parents, as much emotional suppoort as possible should be available.

GRESHAM, F.M.
(1982)
*Exceptional
Children,* 48, 5,
422–33.

Misguided mainstreaming: The case for social skills training with handicapped children

The author reviews some 40 studies (mainly of retarded or maladjusted children) which show that the handicapped child is not generally accepted by his peers in an integrated class. He argues that mainstreaming is not in itself helpful, but that it can be if the handicapped pupil is given social skills training. He discusses research on suitable curricula for social skills training.

HEGARTY, S.,
POCKLINGTON, K.
and LUCAS, D.
(1982)
Windsor: NFER-
Nelson.

Integration in Action

Part of a project on the integration of handicapped pupils into ordinary schools (see also Hegarty *et al.*, 1981). This volume takes 14 integration programmes – for pupils with learning difficulties, with physical handicaps, with impaired hearing and vision, and with speech difficulties – and examines them in detail.

ALSTON, J.
(1983)
Special Education,
10, 4, 19–23.

Children with brittle bones: an examination of their educational needs and progress

The study was carried out in two parts; initially, 20 children aged four to nine with brittle bones were identified and compared with a control group of matched children. On tests of ability the affected children were equal to the non-handicapped children, but there was some evidence that the children in special schools were not doing as well as those in ordinary schools. Additional data from a questionnaire circulated by the Brittle Bone Society suggested that placement in special or ordinary schools was rather arbitrary. In the second stage of the study 40 children with the condition were compared with non-handicapped children on tests of intelligence and literacy; again, overall achievement was similar in the two groups, but the children in special schools were behind the others in reading and writing. Although placement in special schools was related to severer handicap, there were mildly handicapped children in special schools and severely handicapped ones – doing well socially and educationally – in ordinary schools. Those in special schools were not always achieving their full potential, especially in writing.

HODGSON, A.
(1984)
Special Education,
11, 1, 27–9.

Integrating physically handicapped pupils

A brief summary of points taken from the author's book (see Hodgson *et al.*, 1984). Planning is essential to integrating handicapped pupils into ordinary classes. The school should find out as much as possible about the pupil beforehand; decisions should be made about physical adaptations. Support from specialist personnel should be encouraged, and class teachers be prepared to work with welfare assistants and physiotherapists. The limits of the child's mobility and energy should be understood. Seating and special equipment are discussed, and the handling of emergencies. Wherever possible pupils should join in physical education and extracurricular activities.

HODGSON, A.,
CLUNIES-ROSS, L.
and HEGARTY, S.
(1984)
Windsor: NFER-
Nelson.

Learning Together

Seventy-six schools in 21 LEAs in England and Wales were visited by the authors in order to learn how they adapted to teaching handicapped pupils. Twenty-six of them were then chosen for closer study. Aspects of their work that were studied include pupil grouping, organization of supplementary teaching, timetabling, modification of the curriculum, staffing, in-service training, and classroom organization and practice.

SECTION V
General

The majority of articles and books in this section are concerned with the care and management of handicapped children. Only those which deal specifically with orthopaedically handicapped children or which are particularly relevant to their problems and those of their families are included. Other works summarized cover a variety of topics: accounts by parents of orthopaedically handicapped children, experiences of the handicapped themselves and traditional attitudes to the congenitally deformed. For those interested in aspects of orthopaedic disabilities not included in this booklet, such as incidence, epidemiology and physical characteristics, a reference is given to *The Handicapped Child: Research Review,* Vol. II (Dinnage, 1972), which covers sensory and physical handicaps.

WALTON, J.N.
(1965)
New Society,
4 March, 17–18.

Muscular dystrophy and the family

A brief description for the layman of the disease, its effect on the patient and the family, and genetic transmission.

HUNT, P. (Ed)
(1966)
Geoffrey
Chapman.

Stigma. The Experience of Disability

Twelve physically handicapped adults vividly describe their own experience and their relationships with the community.

YOUNGHUSBAND,
E., BIRCHALL,
D.,
DAVIE, R., and
KELLMER
PRINGLE, K.L.
(Eds)
(1970)
London. National
Bureau for Co-
operation in Child
Care.

Living with Handicap

A synopsis of the report of the working party on the needs of handicapped children under the chairmanship of Dame Eileen Younghusband. Evidence and information was obtained from professional and voluntary organizations, local authorities and from parents of handicapped children, and on the basis of these contributions and of their own experience in various disciplines concerned with handicapped children, the 18 members of the working party have made detailed recommendations on every aspect of their subject.

DINNAGE, R.
(1972)
London:
Longman in
association with
the National
Children's
Bureau.

The Handicapped Child: Research Review Vol II

Review of research since 1958, covering sensory and physical handicaps. Selected studies are abstracted and there is a comprehensive annotated bibliography.

DOWNEY, J.A.
and LOW, N.L.
(Eds)
(1974)
W.B. Saunders.

The Child with Disabling Illness

Twenty-seven chapters by American specialists include selected chronic medical illnesses, disorders of the neuromuscular system, disorders of the musculoskeletal system and injuries, and psychosocial aspects.

Section V: *General*

Fox, A.M.
(1974)
London: Camden
and Islington Area
Health Authority.

'They get this training, but they don't really know how you feel'

Nine taped interviews with parents of children with varying handicaps are given verbatim, and many issues important to them are raised.

**Jacobs, J.C. and
Downey, J.A.**
(1974)
In: Downey, J.A.
and Low, N.L.
(Eds) *The Child
with Disabling
Illness.* W.B.
Saunders.

Juvenile rheumatoid arthritis

An outline of symptoms, diagnosis, management and outcome.

**Katz, J.F. and
Challenor,
Y.B.**
(1974)
In: Downey, J.A.
and Low, N.L.
(Eds) *The Child
with Disabling
Illness.* W.B.
Saunders.

Childhood orthopedic syndromes

Descriptions of congenital hip dislocation, Perthes disease, and slipped epiphysis in adolescence.

Myers, S.J.
(1974)
In: Downey, J.A.
and Low, N.L.
(Eds) *The Child
with Disabling
Illness.* W.B.
Saunders.

The spinal injury patient

A description of trauma occurring at birth or due to accidents; patterns of injury, secondary deformities, methods of treatment and psychosocial rehabilitation.

Britton, E.
(1978)
*Educational
Research,* 21, 1,
3–9.

Warnock and integration

In this article based upon a paper read to the Annual Meeting of the British Association for the Advancement of Science, Sir Edward Britton discusses changing attitudes to handicap, challenges the medical model of the handicapped child, and distinguishes between handicap and disability. He examines arguments for and against the new hopes for teaching children together in an integrated setting wherever possible.

GREENBERG, R. (1979) *Adolescent Psychiatry*, 7, 281–8.

Psychiatric aspects of physical disability: impact on the family

The author emphasizes that the disabled should be allowed to express grief over their disabilities if they want to, and to bring up any feelings they may have of envy and bitterness towards the able-bodied.

SPENCER, M. (1980) *Special Education*, 7, 1, 18–20.

Wheelchairs in a primary school

An account by the headteacher of a primary school taking in a large number of children with varied handicaps, and the adaptations and additions required for their needs.

DARNBOROUGH, A. and KINRADE, D. (1981) Cambridge: Woodhead-Faulkner in association with the Royal Association for Disability and Rehabilitation.

Directory for the Disabled

A resource directory of use to all concerned with handicap.

ALSTON, J. (1982) *Special Education*, 9, 2, 29–32.

Children with brittle bones

A description of the cause and signs of this inherited disorder. Children with brittle bones do have normal intelligence; a small sample tested had a mean IQ of 109. Case histories of three children who achieved well in ordinary primary schools are given.

FLETCHER, I. (1982) *Maternal and Child Health*, 7, 12, 490–7.

The management of limb deficient children

The wide variety of limb anomalies are described, and early counselling and referral to an artificial limb and appliance centre recommended. The role of occupational therapists is also very important.

Section V: *General*

MUSCULAR
DYSTROPHY
GROUP OF GREAT
BRITAIN
(1982)

The Muscular Dystrophy Handbook

A comprehensive inventory of medical services, mobility aids, methods of day-to-day management, housing needs, education and training, leisure activities.

PHILP, M. and
DUCKWORTH, D.
(1982)
Windsor: NFER-
Nelson.

Children with Disabilities and their Families: a review of research

All aspects of handicapped children's upbringing – practical problems, parents' adjustment, the social and emotional adjustment of the child, siblings' problems, information and services – are discussed in relation to research findings. Over 200 references are listed.

BEALES, G.
(1984)
Nursing, 2, 3,
908–9.

Juvenile arthritis: the 'whole child' approach

How to treat the patient with juvenile arthritis so that confidence is built up and the child may realize her potential. The illness and the treatments should be fully explained. Outside interests should be encouraged, and parents dissuaded from over-protection.

CHAPLIN, L.
(1984)
Health Visitor, 57,
8, 236–7.

Duchenne muscular dystrophy: a need for awareness

The author highlights the need for a better understanding of the condition and the strains it imposes on the families involved. The importance of early and accurate diagnosis is stressed.

FLETCHER, I.,
CARTWRIGHT, R.,
and ROCKEY, J.
(1984)
In: McCARTHY,
G.T. (Ed) *The
Physically
Handicapped
Child*. London:
Faber and Faber.

Limb deficiency

An outline of the possible conditions and their management.

McCARTHY, G.T. (Ed) (1984) London: Faber and Faber.

The Physically Handicapped Child

Contributors come from the medical, nursing, paramedical, psychological, sociological and educational fields; the emphasis is on practical facts and care. There are chapters on cerebral palsy, spina bifida, arthrogryphosis, limb deficiencies, muscular dystrophy, spinal deformity, head injuries, orthotics, rehabilitation engineering and multidisciplinary assessment.

ROBINSON, A. (1984) London: National Children's Bureau.

Respite Care Services

A National Children's Bureau pamphlet which examines the role of temporary caring services for families with a handicapped child. Types of service available – residential care, family-based care, care in the child's home, holiday schemes – are described, and the factors which contribute towards their success. Staff qualifications, both professional and voluntary, are discussed; research into the subject is reviewed. A list of names and addresses is appended.

ROBINSON, R.O. (1984) In: McCARTHY, G.T. (Ed) *The Physically Handicapped Child*. London: Faber and Faber.

Neuromuscular disorders and muscular dystrophy

A brief account of diagnosis, genetic aspects, symptoms and progress of the condition.

RUSSELL, P. (1984) London: Souvenir Press.

The Wheelchair Child (2nd ed)

A handbook for parents, covering problems from early childhood to young adulthood. Basic information on the main handicapping conditions are included, together with the medical and community services available and much practical advice on aids, appliances, home adaptations and financial grants. The developmental and emotional problems attached to disability are sensitively discussed.

Author Index

Katz, J.F. and Challenor, Y.B. (1974) 49
Kimmel, J. (1959) 15
Kleck, R., Oni, H. and Hastorf, A.H. (1966) 5
Kohlberg, L.J. and Rothenberg, M.B. (1970) 18
Kornfeld, M.S. and Siegel, I.M. (1979) 33
Lambert, C.N., Hamilton, R.C. and Pellicore, R.J. (1969) 18
Lazar, A.L., Gensley, J.T. and Orpet, R.E. (1971) 9
Leibowitz, D. and Dubowitz, V. (1981) 44

McAnarney, E.R., Pless, B., Satterwhite, B. and Friedman, S.B. (1974) 20
McCarthy, G.T. (Ed) (1984) 52
McDaniel, J.W. (1969) 8
McKeever, P.T. (1981) 33
Marsh, G.G. (1972) 38
Marsh, G.G. and Munsat, T.L. (1974) 39
Muscular Dystrophy Group of Great Britain (1982) 51
Myers, S.J. (1974) 49
Myers, B.A., Friedman, S.B. and Weiner, I.B. (1970) 19

Philp, M. and Duckworth, D. (1982) 51
Pless, I.B. and Pinkerton, P. (1975) 21
Pope-Grattan, M.M., Burnett, C.N. and Wolfe, C.V. (1976) 21

Rapier, J., Adelson, R., Carey, R. and Croke, K. (1972) 10
Reite, M., Davis, K., Solomons, C. and Ott, J. (1972) 19
Richardson, S.A. (1970) 8, (1971) 9
Richardson, S.A., Goodman, N., Hastorf. A.H. and Dornbusch, S.M. (1961) 3

Rimon, R., Belmaker, R.H. and Ebstein, R. (1977) 22
Robinson, A. (1984) 52
Rosenbaum, P.L. and Armstrong, R.W. (1984) 12
Russell, P. (1984) 52

Schatzinger, L.A.H., Nash, C.L., Drotar, D.D. and Hall, T.W. (1977) 23
Schechter, M.D. (1961) 15
Schorer, C.E. (1964) 16
Shears, L.M. and Jensema, C.J. (1969) 8
Sherwin, A.C. and McCully, R.S. (1961) 15
Shindi, J. (1983) 27
Siegel, I.M. and Kornfeld, M.S. (1980) 24
Siller, J. and Chipman, A. (1964) 4
Smits, S.J. (1964) 17
Spencer, M. (1980) 50
Standen, P.J. (1983) 27

Tringo, J.L. (1970) 9

Volpe, R. (1976) 21

Walton, J.N. (1965) 48
Weinberg, N. (1978) 11
Wilkinson, V.A. (1981) 24
Worden, D.K. and Vignos, P.J. (1962) 36

Younghusband, E., Birchall, D., Davie, R. and Kellmer Pringle, K.L. (Eds) (1970) 48

Yuker, H.E., Block, J.R. and Young, J.H. (1966 and 1970) 5
Yule, W. and Rutter, M. (1970) 37